Apple Cider Vinegar Health Benefits

35 Suprising Uses

Joanna Aphiah

Apple Cider Vinegar Health Benefits: 35 Surprising Uses by Joanna Aphiah.

Published by Kwizbud Publishing House, 204C Chestnut Crossing Dr.,Newark 19713, New Jersey, U.S.A.

Books@kwizbud.com

Copyright © **2019 Joanna Aphiah**

ISBN: 9781699268117

Table of Contents

PREFACE

Apple cider vinegar, or cider vinegar, as the name implies, is a vinegar made from fermented apple juice. It is made by crushing apples, then fermenting the squeezed out juice. It is used as a food preservative, dressings in salad and other food preparation besides its well known medicinal uses.

Have you tried using apple cider vinegar (ACV) in your salad or drinking it? It is not necessary to consume so much ACV, anyways. 20-30 ml in your salad dressing or your morning water are enough if you desire to use it every day.

Apple cider vinegar is a miracle food with many benefits for our health. However, you should always remember that even the healthiest food can cause harm if you have too much of it. So always consult your doctor first before starting to take any supplements. Apple cider vinegar is highly acidic and can lower potassium levels and bone density. Beware that you can harm your teeth if you drink too much apple cider vinegar over a long period.

This book details the uses of apple cider vinegar in many common day to day applications as well as how to prepare the apple cider vinegar for the various uses.

The history of apple cider vinegar dates back over 5,000 years ago when the Babylonians and Egyptians kept cider vinegar vessels. Later, Hippocrates, the father of modern medicine, treated his patients with apple cider vinegar in 400 B.C. while writing about its health benefits in many of his thesis. Christopher Columbus had it on board his ships to prevent disease, and Julius Caesar's army considered it an essential part of their diet.

Today, apple cider vinegar is sort after the world over by film and music stars and politicians, captains of industry to super moms who care deeply about the health of their families.

Apple Cider Vinegar Health Benefits-35 Surprising Uses presents some fantastic applications of Apple cider vinegar in a fun way. The book also shares a variety of recipes to help you discover the true path to health and a long, happy life.

Joanna Aphiah

I adopted a healthier diet. I take at least a tablespoon of apple cider vinegar a day. It's an old wives' tale, but it is one of the best things you can put in your mouth.

-Melissa Etheridge

We stopped cleaning our homes with lemon water, and cider vinegar like our mothers did, and now we clean with chemicals. We're inhaling chemicals, and then everyone wonders why cancer is the biggest killer.

-Suzanne Somers

How to Take Apple Cider Vinegar

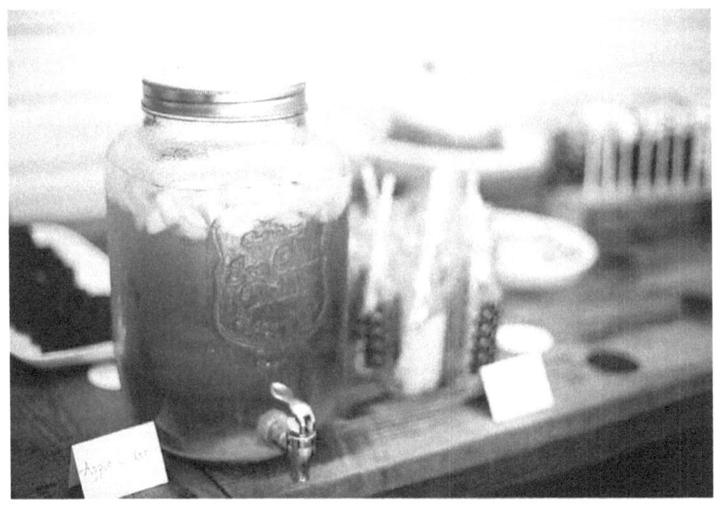

Many people know the uses of apple cider vinegar for food. However, all over the globe, there are some unknown and over-looked uses we shall quickly add here.

Despite the numerous qualities of Apple Cider Vinegar, it has an awful taste, and this could have an opposite effect for some people. So if you are a lover of Apple Cider Vinegar, adding water to the solution will be a good choice. If the taste is still discouraging, use fresh honey to dilute it.

Diarrhea Treatment

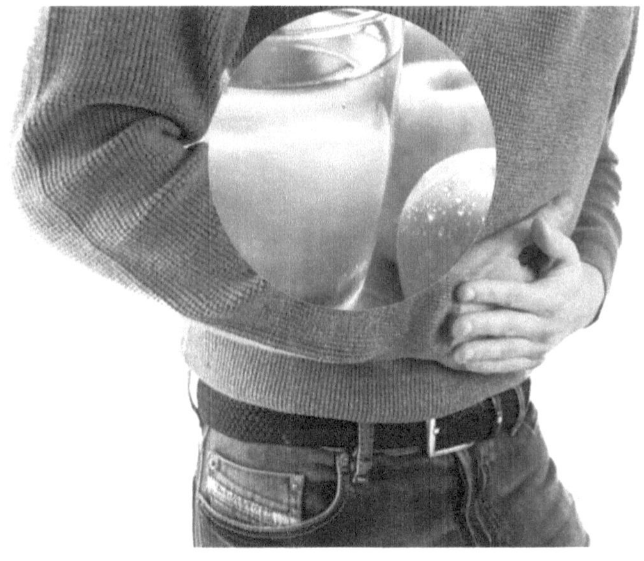

Apple cider vinegar contains a special element called pectin that helps treat diarrhea by forming large fibrous matter. This serves as a layer of coat that protects and helps keep your gut safe.

How to use

Mix one or two tablespoons of apple cider vinegar in water. Drink twice daily for two days or until symptom stops.

Indigestion Cure

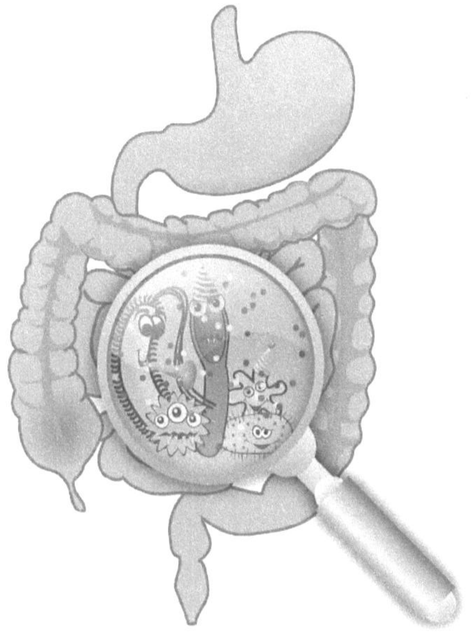

If you are eating less fibrous food, you need to take a cup of the apple cider vinegar syrup before eating.

How to use:

Add one teaspoon of honey and one teaspoon
apple cider vinegar to a cup of warm water.

Stuffy Nose Treatment

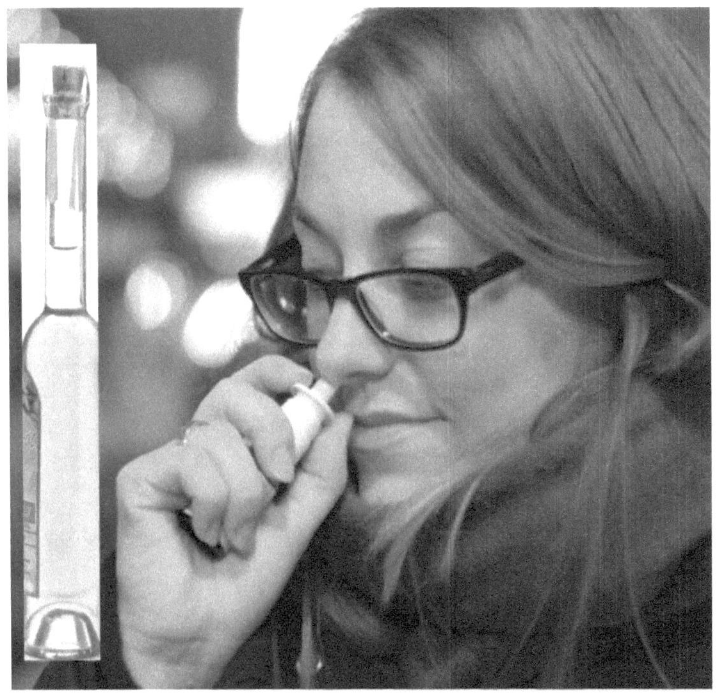

Do you have a stuffy nose? Or you need help stopping running nose?

How to use

Mix a teaspoon of apple cider vinegar in a cup of water and drink. Take this twice a day until symptom disappears.

Sore throat Treatment

A sore throat could affect how we talk among our colleague and friends. When you notice this, for those having a sore throat, you will get relief soon enough when you take the apple cider vinegar. And it helps inhibit the multiplication of most germs due to its acidic nature.

How to use

Mix up one-quarter (¼) cup apple cider vinegar with ¼ cup warm water and take a sip every sixty minutes till the sore feeling ends.

Stress Relief

Stress may cause a buildup of lactic acid in your body. When you are tired and need some rest, apple cider vinegar can be of great help because of the potassium enzymes present in it.

How to use

Add a tablespoon or two of apple cider vinegar to a glass of chilled vegetable drink or to a glass of water. Take for two days.

Bad Breath Remedy

Does having bad breath make you feel ashamed or shy?

How to use

Add ½ tablespoon of ACV into a cup of water and take a sip, hold for some time in your mouth and gaggle then pour it out. Do not drink it. Observe what happens after some days.

Fight Yeast Infections

Use in treating yeast infection. A common yeast infection is the vagina yeast infection caused by the fungus Candida. This infection can cause intense itchiness, inflammation and a thick white discharge in the case of the vagina.

How to use

Add one and a half-cup of ACV into a Bathroom tub filled with warm water, allow it to dissolve for about 20 minutes. Do this once every day for the first three days.

Foot or Skin Fungus Application

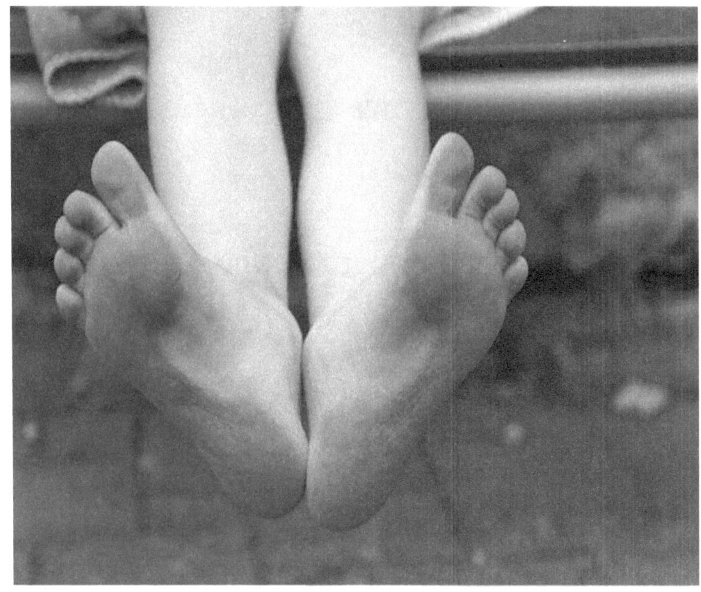

Do you have any yeast infections on any part of your body? Then the apple cider vinegar can help in killing infections on your skin and nails.

How to use

Set a bucket of water and put your feet in a cup of ACV in water.

You may also apply some to the affected area. When you are treating skin fungus or yeast, apply directly

When you have a situation where the skin is sensitive, there is every need to dilute it before applying to the area.

Reduce blood sugars.

It has some anti-glycemic effects that boost insulin sensitivity, and this helps to control the level of blood sugar in the body.

How to use

Mix one teaspoon of Apple Cider Vinegar in a glass of clean water and take it three times a day, so your stomach is prepared. This will regulate your sugar levels. Go for medical advice if you are diabetic.

Rapid Weight Loss

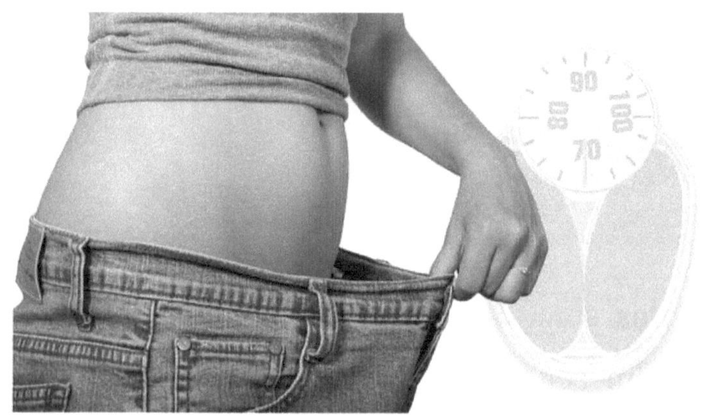

Apple Cider Vinegar helps in reducing weight when it speeds up fat loss process.

How to use

Pour two teaspoons of the vinegar into a cup of water and drink before eating, or you may drink it slowly to see greater results.

Hair Wash

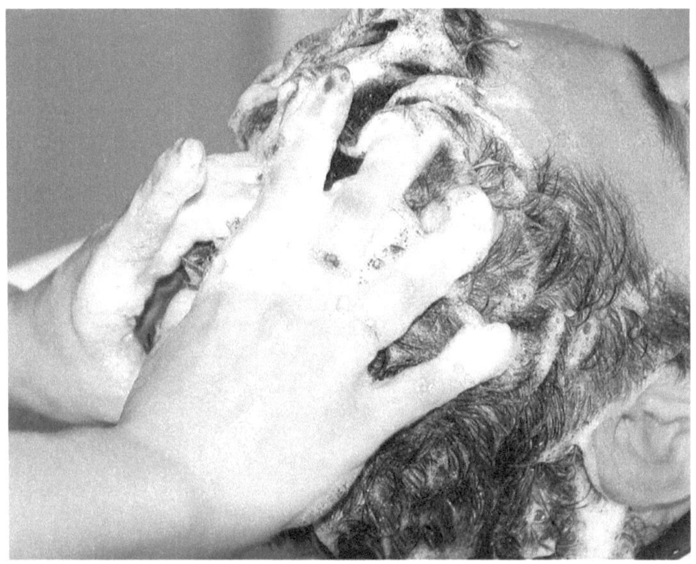

Acetic acid is one of the acids that helps hair shine. Quantities of this acid are present in ACV, and you can use the apple cider vinegar to cleanse your hair the PH level constant. Clears away every form of dandruff

How to use

Mix 1/3 cup ACV in 4 cups of water and wash hair with the mixture. Allow for some time after using shampoo before rinsing.

Facial Mask Application

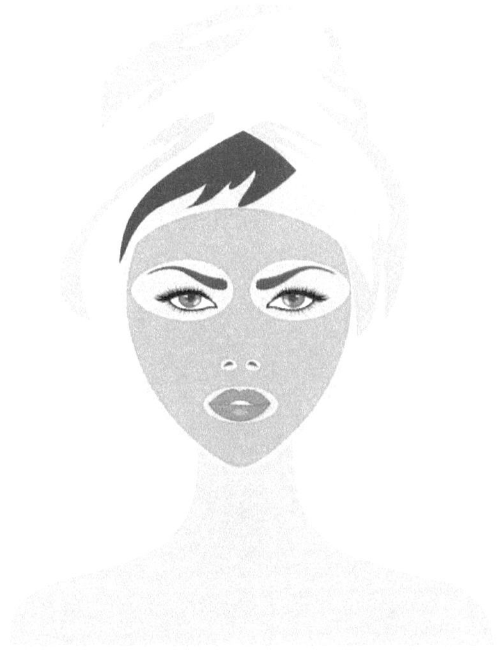

Face mask are also an excellent way to pull out impurities, hydrate the skin, remove excess oils and improve the appearance of your pores.

How to use

Combine equal parts apple cider vinegar and bentonite clay, add one tablespoon of honey. Apply them on your skin and allow for some time about ten to fifteen minutes. After this, rinse off.

Blemishes Minimization

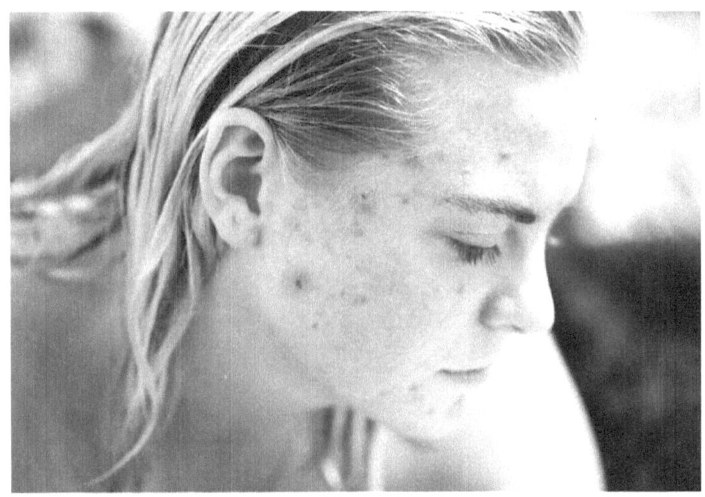

Yes, Apple cider vinegar can be used for inflammation purposes. Do you have any inflammation on your skin? Then try using the ACV

How to use

Using a cotton bud, dip it in dilute apple cider vinegar liquid and rub on the affected areas. Leave for some minutes and wash off

Soothing Bath Soak

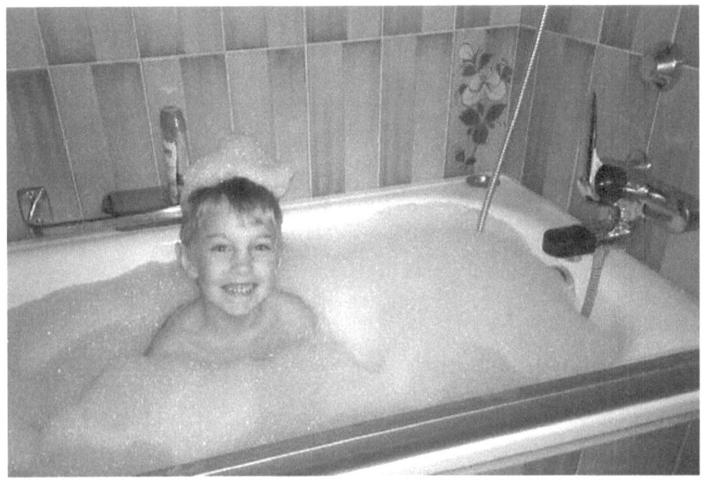

To deal with skin rashes, irritations or you just want to have a warm bath, apply the ACV.

How to use

Add one to two capfuls of apple cider vinegar

in your water, and use to bath. It removes toxins out of the body, making your skin toned and moisturized skin.

Teeth Whitener

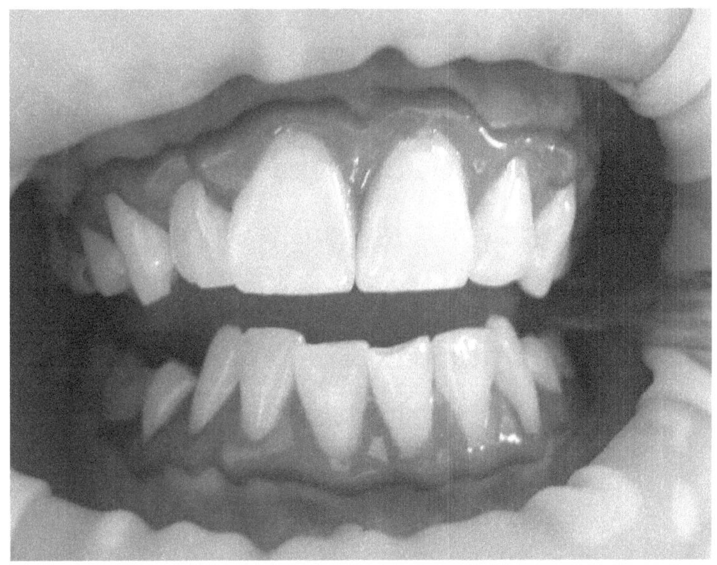

Its acid properties make it effective against bacteria and germs. it is used in some quarters to remove teeth stains.

How to use

Take a sip very early in the morning when you are about going to brush your teeth. Gargle it for some time and pour it out.

Rub a small amount of apple cider vinegar onto your teeth with a cotton pad. Do this repeatedly, and with time the stains will clear away. Be careful, though as you should wash when done with plenty of water. You don't want to allow it acidic nature to affect your enamel.

Skin Peeling Remedy

Do you have sunburn or is any part of your skin peeling off?

How to use

Ease your pain applying a washcloth soaked in apple cider vinegar to the area.

Age-Spots Reduction

Apple Cider Vinegar helps you fight against germs and other fungi due to its possession of Sulphur.

How to use

Now for you to use it for this purpose, rub on the affected area where you have the dark spot. Leave overnight and wash off early in the morning.

Varicose Vein Treatment

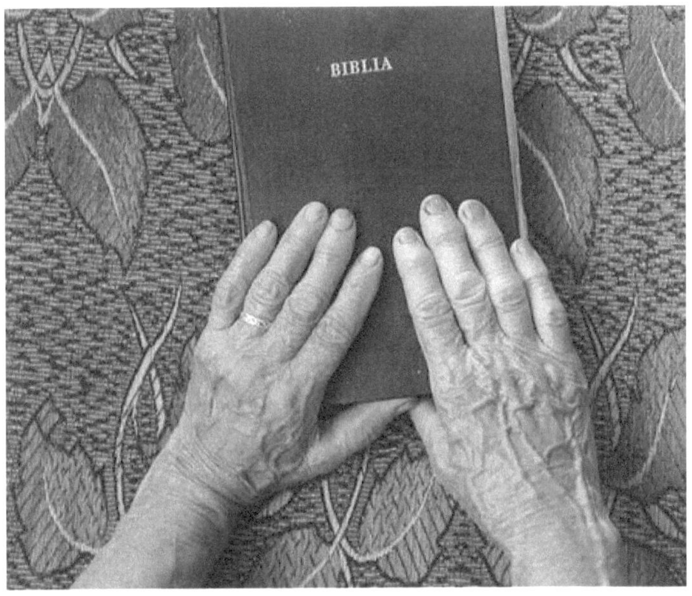

Apple cider vinegar is great for treating varicose veins. This vein helps your body vessels and transmits blood. To improve circulation, follow the process below.

How to use

Pour some on the area where you have the varicose vein. Massage gently with a washcloth. Repeat every day continuously for 21 days. You will see improvement in blood circulation.

Natural Deodorant

Deodorants that are sold commercially can limit your ability to sweat greatly. It's been confirmed that sweating is the body's natural way of detoxification. So the apple cider vinegar can be used as a natural deodorant. It absorbs and neutralizes odors.

How to use

Pour some on a soft cloth and rub the underarms. The smell disappears when it's dried up.

.

Wart Removal

They are caused by the human papilloma virus (HPV). They are harmless raised bumps on the hands and feet.

How to use

Mix two parts apple cider vinegar in one-part water.

Soak a cotton pad in apple cider vinegar, put it on the wart and hold tightly with a bandage. Leave It till next day. Repeat this process for one week.

Arthritic Pain Remedy

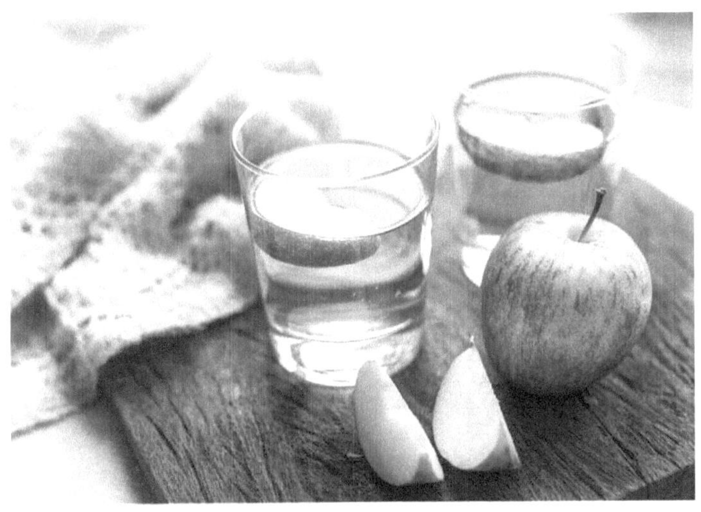

The apple cider vinegar contains potassium which works to prevent calcium build-up in the joints, which causes joint stiffness and arthritis pain.

How to use

To use, get a soft cloth and dip in ACV liquid, gently massage over the area. Repeat the process at least thrice a day till relief is achieved.

Body Fluid Regulation

For daily maintenance of the numan body electrolyte, weight loss, and pH balancing; Apple Cider Vinegar could be used effectively.

How to use

Take two teaspoons in 200ml of water thrice a day especially before you eat any food

Acid Reflux, Cough, or Bronchitis Remedies

Common symtoms of cold can be relieved by the intake of Apple Cider Vineger

How to use

Take two tablespoons in 200ml of water thrice a day. Do this before eating.

Apple Cider Vinegar Detox

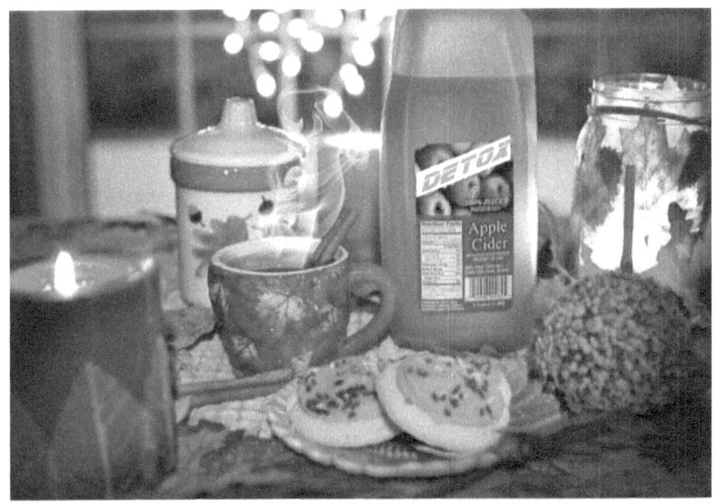

The apple cider vinegar is a natural acid. Yes, it's acidic in nature, so it is always advisable to dilute it in water before taking it or using it for body detox.

Wash your mouth with water after each detox. Drink with a straw if necessary.

Apple cider vinegar may also interact with different medications, consult your doctor before you start using apple cider vinegar regularly or try the detox.

Some patients mentioned that using ACV has caused nausea or stomach discomfort, especially when the stomach is empty.

Trying an apple cider vinegar detox is likely safe for most people.

There are places where it's used majorly as an apple cider vinegar detox.

The idea of the detox is using raw, unfiltered apple cider vinegar which still has "the mother" in it. It's believed to contain vitamins and essential minerals that are useful for this purpose, although it may sometimes look cloudy. For thousands of years, many have known and used the ACV for detoxification purposes.

When you plan on introducing a new diet or change from one diet program to another, you may choose to detoxify. Here are some important facts:

Source of a good body of enzymes

Supporting a healthy immune system from its calcium component

Effective in weight control

Maintain proper PH

aiding with healthy digestion

adding good bacteria for the gut and immune function

It removes harmful toxins from the body

It causes a soothing effect on the skin

It cures acne.

How to use

1. One or two tablespoons of raw, unfiltered apple cider vinegar

2. Eight ounces of purified or distilled water

3. One to two tablespoons sweetener (organic honey, or maple syrup, or four drops of Stevia)

We have so many variations of this drink. Some of them may add lemon juice.

When you want to do an apple cider vinegar drink detox, follow it through for a week or for several days until a month. Give it time to see potential results with it.

You may decide to take it three times a day.

Acne Remedy

Apple cider vinegar helps kills bacteria and balances skin's pH level. Different things cause acne, but the chief of this is excessive oils.

Since it's a natural acid, apple cider vinegar should be diluted before it's applied to the skin. Here are some simple steps you can follow:

How to use

Mix 1 part apple cider vinegar with 3 three parts water (you may add more water if you want).

Clean your face and use a soft cloth to dry it.

Apply the mix with a cotton cloth. Allow it to stay for 30 seconds. Then rinse and dry.

Repeat this process three times a week

You may also try using the mother with it. The mother is the ACV mixture that has a partial cloudy appearance. It possesses enzymes with so many health benefits.

Apple cider vinegar should be diluted with water before being applied to the skin.

All-Purpose Cleaner

Apple cider vinegar can kill bacteria to some extent. Clean all your dishes with this. It helps kills germs and bacteria

How to use

When you mix it in water, you now have an all-purpose cleaning agent. This cleaning agent is good. Although it doesn't kill all bacteria, it's a sure way to reduce and get rid of bacteria that affect most household things.

You can add ½ cup of apple cider vinegar in water, to make a solvent for washing dishes and more.

Trap Fruit Flies

Fruit flies are major farm and garden pest.

We can use our apple cider vinegar to make a quickly improvised fruit fly trap.

How to use

Pour some apple cider vinegar into a cup, add a few drops of dish soap (to help sink any fly that passes) and place where the flies are constituting a nuisance.

Weeds Killer

Can be used as a homemade weed killer. Weeds are usually a nuisance and can really hinder the growth of choice crops and flowers.

Here's how to do this right away

How to use

Get spraying can. Pour some apple cider vinegar in it. Spray undiluted vinegar on unwanted weeds in your garden to get rid of them. Also, try adding soap or lemon to it.

Alcohol Substitute

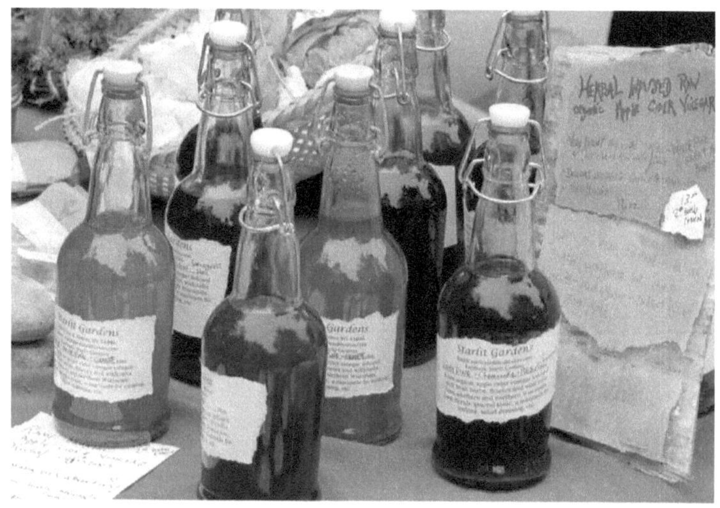

This is useful for people living with alcoholism that are seeking to become sober. How do we achieve this?

How to use

Mix 2 tablespoons of apple cider vinegar, One teaspoon of cinnamon, one tablespoon of honey and two tablespoons of lemon juice into 12 oz (355 ml) of hot water for an alternative hot drink.

Toothbrush Cleaner

Your toothbrush is very vital if you must sustain white and glowing teeth.

Due to its antibacterial properties, the apple cider vinegar can be a cleaner of your toothbrush. Here how.

How to use

To prepare the cleaner, mix half a cup (120 ml) of water with two tablespoons (30 ml) of apple cider vinegar and two teaspoons of baking soda and combine. Dip the head of your brush in the mix and allow to settle there for thirty minutes.

Rinse toothbrush properly with lots of water before using again.

Remove Fleas on Pets

Apple cider vinegar may help prevent your pet from getting fleas.

How to use:

Combine 1 part water and 1 part apple cider vinegar and mix thoroughly. Using a soft cloth or cotton pad dip in apple cider vinegar, rub the affected skin areas of your pet..

Swelling Reduction

Swelling happens when a part of the body is unusually increased due to some underlying factors.

How to use:

Apply some apple cider vinegar and rub the affected swollen hands or feet. This can be useful for pregnant women who sometimes experience swelling feet.

Repel Pussy Cats

You can use Apple Cider Vinegar to prevent unwanted animals from intruding into your environment. Not everyone wants cats around and if you are one of those, you can use ACV {apple cider vinegar) to repel them. Cats hate the smell of ACV

How to use

Mix ACV with water and spray it around to stop cats from intruding..

Aids Sleep

The amino acids in Apple Cider Vinegar help to combat fatigue and has been used as a remedy for insomnia for centuries.

How to Use

You can make a drink by taking a teaspoon of Apple Cider Vinegar and teaspoon of honey and mixing it with warm water. Drink in the evening before you go to bed.

Treats Ear Infections

ACV can help clear up ear infections which cause mild pains or irritation.

How to use

Mix 1 part ACV with 1 part water. Gently use a dropper to apply a few drops into the ear being careful not to force anything into the ear canal.

www.ingramcontent.com/pod-product-compliance
Lightning Source LLC
Chambersburg PA
CBHW051230250726
48655CB00006B/2701